I0440546

Weight Loss Inspiration

Step by Step Methods to Successfully Lose Weight

JANE JOHN-NWANKWO RN, MSN

Jane John-Nwankwo RN, MSN

Weight Loss Inspiration:
Step by Step Methods to Successfully Lose Weight

Copyright © 2014 by Jane John-Nwankwo.

All rights reserved. No part of this book may be reproduced or transmitted in any form or by any means without written permission from the author.

ISBN-13: 978-1499377903

ISBN-10: 1499377908

Printed in the United States of America

Dedication

Dedicated to all who wish to lose 10, 20, 30, 100, 200

or any amount of pounds. You can make it work!

OTHER TITLES FROM THE SAME AUTHOR:

1. Hightime you made a move!

2. Accept challenges

3. Never be intimidated

4. Design your own methods to navigate

5. Success is for the ready

6. How to market a website

7. How to start your own business

8. How to make money online with no money

Have you bought these books?

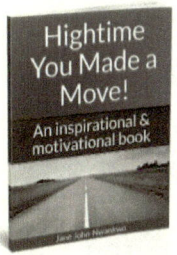 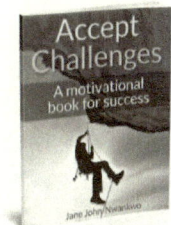 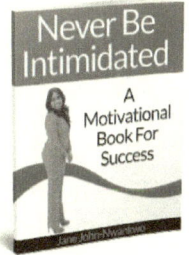

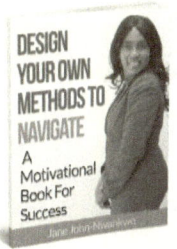 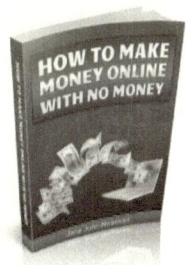 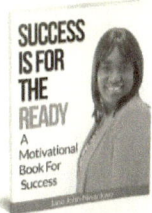

Weight Loss is not about
starvation, It is about eating
the same things you love in
really lesser quantities.
Discipline!
-Jane John-Nwankwo

Introduction:

Being overweight does not only give you problems towards your own self but the bigger picture is how people look at you while you're out walking on the streets.

The uncomfortable knocking together of your thighs, losing your good old clothes, looking at yourself in the mirror and thinking "When did this all happen?", and many more uncomfortable emotional feelings can be reversed.

Weighing more than your body is allowed to carry makes you look bloated here and there and this may give you some embarrassing situations that often lead to ridicule!

Among the effective ways are: to decide to undergo some form of body renovation by means of exercise, curbing your cravings on food or meeting with a health professional who can give you useful suggestions. There are various measures to help you take off these unsightly excesses; nevertheless, there are also plenty of risks that you have to take and sacrifices to make.

Reading this book without practicing what it says would be like smiling to someone in the dark. If you are ready to go on this self-changing journey, let's go!

You can see all my books at my website:

www.janejohn-nwankwo.com

Chapter 1
Coping with Overweight Issues

This book is not only for overly over-weight people. It is for everyone who would like to lose any amount of pounds. Do you want to go back to size 8 from size 10? This book is for you. Do you wish to go back 5 sizes down? This book is also for you.

Do not procrastinate any longer!

Procrastination is an almost certain way to ensure we don't succeed. There is no better way to throw a well-laid plan off the road to success. We are all guilty at one time or another of procrastinating. I procrastinate over doing my school work—until it is few hours to the deadline. Yet, I am efficient about completing most other tasks. It's easier to put things off than it is to actually get to work on them. Why do we procrastinate even when it is something we want to achieve or know we need to do?

Procrastinators shoot themselves in the foot. They set up road blocks just by putting things off until it is too late to achieve success. Consciously or subconsciously, they make choices that hurt their performance. Consider what time of the year it is now, and think of something you have been desiring to achieve for the past 10 months, but have been putting it off. Can you believe it is ten months already?

Coping with being overweight can be a daunting task. It leads the dieter into creating something that is quite frustrating that at times they would just leave the program they have started. Finding their way back into the same issue is very much possible. Nonetheless, one may find it easier if there are some friends around who can offer good suggestions when it comes to losing unwanted weight that causes disappointments to the person. There are ways to help you go through the feelings that are incurred when overweight issues grow bigger and heavier to bear.

Being antagonistic
Teenagers who are overweight choose to isolate themselves from others who have fit bodies as they become more conscious of how they look like. This may lead them to frustration as other people their age can perform tasks and go into activities that they themselves cannot perform well due to the extra load they carry. Emotional buildup can pave the way to disliking social gatherings in order to avoid being ridiculed by their peers. Sometimes, overweight individuals may become antagonistic towards their friends.

Low performance
Once you know that you are weighing way above normal, you may feel a bit tired most of the time and there would be instances when you would fall asleep as others are enjoying chatting with each other. This is true also on the workplace. While your fellow workers are into some tasks just like you, you would have the tendency to take rests in between that leads you to not finishing the jobs assigned to you within the day; performance at work is lower than that of the more active workers.

Recognizing what you are feeling

Being heavy for your body build is not ultimately bad and you don't have to think about it all the time. Unless you want to stay that way, you had better thought of giving yourself time to plan about how to solve the problem. Never listen to unpleasant remarks. You have to get over with the fact that you are not at all pleased by the way you look. Instead of giving thought to what other people would say to you, why not pick yourself up and make plans to get a better image of you. This way, you can regain your confidence.

Overweight Woes Lead to Frustration
We all know that being overweight takes a lot of thinking and time for us to consider how to shave off those excess pounds. Unwanted fats that grow all over our figure may be the start of an everlasting dilemma that leads to frustration in the long run.
Being overweight does not only give you problems towards your own self but the bigger picture is how people look at you while you're out walking on the streets. This may sound very common but weighing more than your body is allowed to carry makes you look bloated here and there and this may give you some embarrassing situations that often lead to ridicule!

Among the effective ways are to decide to undergo some form of body renovation by means of exercise, curbing your cravings on food or meeting with a health professional who can give you working suggestions. There are various measures to help you take off these unsightly excesses; nevertheless, there are also plenty of risks that you have to take and sacrifices to make.

No exercise routine can be effective if a person is not that bent on doing it religiously. Indeed, there are plenty of these regimens that exercise gurus may suggest to you. However, your regimen must also complement the type of body you have. Fitness instructors must consider the time you can spend on the routine; otherwise, the program may not be effective at all.

Exercise alone can never make your fats go away. Food intake must also be considered by the person aiming to lose weight. There are many diet programs that can go alongside with a specific exercise program and this is what you need to find out. You may visit a certified nutritionist or fitness gym where you can find people who can draft a certain program for you that may include fitness and diet all at the same time.

What your Friends Say about you can hurt you
It is true that not all people know how obesity can damage the self-esteem of an overweight person. People whom you have known for a long time may be the persons who can offer you better advices. So, you better know whom you are talking to regarding the weight issues you have grown to hate. As it takes so much practice in order for you to recognize the kind of feeling you have, never forget that only level-headedness can help you with this dilemma.

In their effort to make you understand that you have gone overboard normal food intake, some of them may say things that could insult you. This is not a good idea at all; friends who know you from head to foot know which word to say and know the right adjective to describe how they feel towards what you are into. You may listen to the bad comments but never forget that truth sometimes could hurt you as a person. Nevertheless, you must listen to every word that is hurled towards you but take only the good ones. It is also helpful not to try being antagonistic, just to cover your self- pride.

If you are able to convert the insults into something that can help motivate you more, then, the better for you to cope with your present situation. There could be no other factor that could propel you towards your aim other than yourself. Therefore, you can listen to bad comments regarding your being overweight and laugh it off when you arrive home. Those words which could have crushed you might just be the wakeup call you need to further strive to get to where you want to be.

Your case may be a worst one but if you can come to focus your attention, you may just be another success story that other people may read on the net! Why waste your time showing off to individuals who have sent you negative remarks when you can satisfy yourself by slowly learning the ropes towards an effective exercise and diet program? There is nobody that would wish you more luck than your own self and much more—you are the sole beneficiary of your renewed person!

Do not be a Procastinator!

The world of the procrastinator

Psychologists say that twenty percent of any group is made up of chronic procrastinators. For them, procrastination is a way of life. They are late to work or to school *because* of traffic. They don't pay their rent on time *because* they received their paycheck late. They're late arriving at church *because* they wanted to sleep late on a weekend. They are always the last ones to hand in their reports *because* of computer problems. One parent joked that her son would be late for his own funeral.

Because of their procrastination, they miss out of getting tickets to a concert, dinner reservations, and tea times. Their gift cards are never redeemed and their email remains unanswered. Chronic procrastinators are the ones who go Christmas shopping on Christmas Eve, buy the Thanksgiving turkey the morning it is to be cooked, and pick up flowers for their mother from a roadside vendor on Mother's Day morning.

In some societies, like Japan and China, procrastination is viewed as a major character flaw and an embarrassment to the family. In North America we see it as a personality quirk. That's why stores in North America stay open until midnight on Christmas Eve, some even open on Christmas morning, stores carry unfrozen turkeys, and those roadside flower vendors do so well. We're too tolerant of procrastinators to lecture them!

Those who try to "fix" a procrastinator start by trying to build time management skills. Procrastination is not a problem of lack of time management. Nor is it the result of poor planning. Procrastinators do not lack the ability to estimate how much time things will take to get done.

It can be said that aiming for weight loss is not an easy job for most, especially for people who lack the motivation to follow even the simplest regimen. Motivation, indeed, proves to be one of the most common problems dieters encounter as programs need to be followed to the dot otherwise, not much can be achieved from any action plan.

Your work needs you to be there and there's a specific time involved; this is easy as long as you will not do overtime. However, when it comes to the home, there are many things to do that require your attention. There may be some emergencies for your family members or your pets to attend to. Bills may pile up once you have not the time to pay them on time. A scheduled house renovation may take more than your days off to see through.

Will you still have the time to insert a couple of hours for an exercise regimen? Where will you insert time for you to prepare for your own diet meal then? If you are good at time management, then, you may be ready to take up extra effort for your body project. I believe that I have control over my time because it is my schedule. If I have to keep up few hours late to accomplish the goal of the day, then, so be it, but keeping late hours habitually is not healthy. Sometimes, however, it is inevitable.

Honestly speaking, your mindset is the element when it comes to shaving pounds off from your body. You may never achieve the right weight once you feel that you cannot do it.

Your thinking and picturing how you would look once this is achieved would go a long way in helping you.

You need to go back to ground zero once you were not able to cope up with the routines. Therefore, you have to put extra effort to make things work out right for you.

Put off the blunder-bearing extra-curricular activities that you can do without as there are no instant results but only instant cooperation on your part as the weight loss subject.

How to Keep yourself Motivated

Motivation is what drives us to commit good performance and it is the thing that makes us stay on a certain project longer than we expect to be into. Without the drive to solve an issue, one can never obtain a solution that's why there has to be proper mind set when going on a plan to solve something.

Losing weight, as an example, is among the problems that need us to have motivation within ourselves. Once motivated, the mind must maintain the aim in order to get to the target fast. If you have the ability to set your eyes on your goal and able to sustain the need for you to make it work, no problems may arise in the process.

Here are some steps that you can use to further motivate yourself on your goal:

Focus

Once you have set your eyes on your goal, let nothing deter you from deviating from it. Focus is what every dieter needs and this may take time for others to achieve. As long as they see the foods they like that have given them those bulges, they would continue to drool and this paves the way to eating excessive amounts of food again.

Eliminate negative feelings

Negative feelings that may arise along the process to lose weight must be eliminated. You may commit blunders once you dwell on what you think is impossible.

Being positive that you can do it may give you more reasons to overcome fears. Never forget that every step you take involves risks. Once you have jumped over this stage, you can get past the negative emotions and eventually, you can get near your target.

Maintain drive

Some dieters would also have a problem maintaining their will to continue on what they have started. After several days or weeks on the program, they find themselves embroiled in some kinds of situation wherein they are no longer determined to finish their mission. When this happens, there is a great chance of falling back into the same trap which is a body full of fats and total disappointment would surface. One way of changing this scenario is to do the program with a friend to make each day of workout or dieting become more enjoyable.

Associate with people who have the traits you'd like to possess.

Choose to form relationships with people who have a positive influence on your behaviors. Identify the people/friends/colleagues/relatives that energize you and bring out the best in you.

Take a page from AA

Alcoholics Anonymous has taught us the importance of having someone to turn to when we feel we are sliding away from where we want   to go with our goals.

Choose someone with his/her own set of goals. Hold each other accountable to your goals and plans. While it's not necessary for both of you to have the same goals, it'll be even better if that's the case! Then you can learn from each other. It's always good to be accountable.

Verbalize your goals.

Tell others about your goals. Listen to what they sound like. Do they sound good? Does that goal roll pleasingly off your tongue? How do you feel when you say it? What are people's reactions?

Often our goals play around in our heads like fantasies. Once we actually say them out loud, things change. We've made a commitment to our goals, ourselves. Those goals become tangible. People don't laugh. Instead they ask how things are coming along. They may even offer resources or support. It's also a great way to keep yourself accountable to your plans.

Find a Mentor

Seek out someone who has already achieved what you hope to accomplish. Seeing actual proof that your goals are very achievable if you take action is one of the best inspirations for action. "If he can do it, I can too."

Restate your dreams.

If you have been procrastinating for a long time over starting losing those excess fats or finally writing that novel or going back to school to achieve your dream career, you might want to restate or "fine tune" your outcome.

What exactly do you want to achieve? What should you do to get there? What are the steps to take? Does your current situation align with that? If it doesn't, what can you do about it? The goal of this book is to impact your life. Even if you are not a chronic procrastinator, you will be honest to say that you procrastinate returning phone calls, or simple things. Whenever you are tempted to procrastinate again, remember that It's HIGHTIME YOU MADE A MOVE! And really It is time to move those fats out of your body!!

Face reality and stop hiding behind excuses.

Are you waiting for a perfect time to start going to the gym or to start cooking healthy meals yourself? There will never be a perfect time! You will always be able to find excuses to hide behind. Ditch those excuses. If you keep waiting for one, you are never going to achieve that dream!

Get organized. Create a roadmap to success.

One way to commit to that first step in reaching your dream is to create a game plan. Write a detailed timeline. Include specific deadlines. If all you have is an end-goal, that's like handing a procrastinator a "procrastinate forever" card.

Having no set dates for steps along the path to the gold at the end of the rainbow almost assures you will never arrive at that pot of gold. Creating a master timeline with specific tasks along the path is a roadmap to success. As you reach each task and check it off, it empowers you to continue.

What you've done is create an urgency to act. Goals can be broken down into monthly, weekly, and even daily task lists. That list is a call to action. You must accomplish this by the specified date. Otherwise, your goals will be delayed or jeopardized.

Chapter 2
Preparing to Solve the Problem

Preparing to solve the problem of being overweight is easy once you have found yourself armed with the right frame of mind and have the decision to go with a particular program. You may need to prep yourself up with the things you need and knowing where to go for help can allow you more chances of staying put with the goal itself. There are some things that can remind you your target weight and below are some of them:

- Assessing yourself: Take time to assess how you feel towards your weight. Ask yourself what you have been eating in the recent months and why you have grown fond of that food. At one time, I found myself eating lots of ice cream. It gradually became a habit. I packed assorted kinds of it and ate it with my children. When that set finished, I purchased more. Within 3 months, I added about 15 pounds. That was not funny because I quickly moved up a size. The solution was simple: I stopped buying ice cream. I also reduced my juice intake. I drank lots of water and within 6 months. I lost 10 pounds. I did not work out. If I had, I sure would have lost that weight faster. Recognizing your 'temptation food' is one of the keys to losing your weight.

Do you take meals on an irregular basis? If that is so, then, you have a problem. Sometimes we tend to skip meals in order to finish the task we are at and this leads to overindulgence once we are free from work. Skipping breakfast has been scientifically proven to make people add weight. That was one of the first surprises I learnt in nursing school. Always have a little breakfast. It gets your body going in the right direction.

- Curbing your emotions: Know how to cut back your emotions and you should never hate yourself for what you have become. If you have grown fat, well, there are still people who love you for just being you.

  Never think that some of them hate you just because your body was blown out of proportion. All you need is a little time thinking over what you have done in the past and prepare to avoid them voluntarily.

- Dealing with tension the right way: Stress can give you a great time to eat; or haven't you noticed it? Haven't you found your eating habits change once you are preparing for something important? For other people, eating would be less. But for those who have slow metabolism, weight may add up and provide them with rounder and heavier figure.

Eating should be enjoyable but to a certain extent. Know your limits once you take in more food in one meal.

Taking in much more than your body is allowed to take leads to weight gain.

Let me tell you a bit about how the stomach is made up. The stomach is like a balloon. It has stretchable muscles in it known as the stomach *Ruggae*. The stomach ruggae can be trained, but only to a certain extent. When we regularly eat small amounts of food, the stomach stays the same; When we eat a little bit more once in a while, it stretches to accommodate it, then retracts back to our original quantities. But if we maintain the more quantities, the ruggae gradually loses its retractability, and so you have to eat to that amount to satisfy your hunger.

If you add more quantities, it stretches more and remains stretched, it can no longer go back to its original state. Any wonder why you have to eat more now than you did many months ago? Because you have trained your stomach to eat more and your hunger is not quenched until you fill it up. As far you are not overly over-weight, you can still retrain your stomach. It is only when the stomach has lost its retractability that an individual would require a gastric-reduction surgery.

Now that you are prepared for your weight loss program, you are now expected to take the risks that go with it. Among the many risks that you have to face is changing your lifestyle and changing your eating habits.

Let us not forget that we must have a budget that goes with our selected program and that is what we also have to prepare for. When I say budget, I don't necessary mean spending more. I inclusion of healthier foods like fruits and vegetables, instead of other unhealthy stuff you have been used to.

Planning to take on some kind of exercise program involves a budget and this may cost you some $20 a month. Budget for fitness is different from the budget that you may spend on your diet meals which is required to complement your fitness routine. As I have said, it is not a budget that will break the back. There are special meals that you can use and you have to buy all the ingredients.

Exercise regimens may also include the length of time you have to spend on a particular fitness gym to tune up some of your body parts. Sparing some time for your new routine can take away some of your time with your loved ones. However, this sacrifice is the thing that matters most as even though you are capable of paying for your fitness instructor and able to buy diet meals, time is an essential part of your program. Spending time that is needed for your aim can make all of your dreams come true.

Everybody loves food but taking excessive amounts of it can damage not only your health but your self-esteem. Illnesses can be derived from overeating and you can be a subject of ridicule once you can no longer walk normally due to being overweight and fitting into clothes that you used to wear makes you look like a clown. Therefore, if you are targeting a particular weight, cut down on your extra chows and gets a diet plan to make it work.

Getting into the right mind set can get your goal going and going for the betterment of your physical appearance. Once you have prepared to undergo a particular diet plan, your body and mind would come together to start doing their own thing. It would be up to you if you know how to balance the act to make it beneficial for you.

The mind works over matter. Therefore, if you are aiming to lose some weight, everything would come from the mind before the real action, as done by the body, can be put it into fruition. So, if there were a lot of times when you have tried to curb your eating habits and did some exercise for just a short time then stopped; it may be the work of being unable to control yourself mentally.

The brain is the one that dictates on the body. The body reciprocates by putting the mental task to action and the benefits are really good! What other people do is to think about achieving something the fast way; there is no faster way than knowing how to control your body by means of your brain. Once the brain sends out the necessary task, the body goes with what is being dictated.

Following a targeted weight is easy once you have gotten used to avoiding habits that may get you back to your old heavy self. Even if you are the best tactician in mind conditioning, nothing can beat a deadly sight of a sumptuous meal or a mouth-watering cake! Of course, there are people who cannot perform exercise anymore, like those who have previous brushes with accidents.

If some parts of your leg were joined together by metal, then, there is no way for you to get into some rigid routines but you can still perform routines that would not involve severe exercises. You may ask a certified therapist or a fitness expert to draft a softer approach that can make you lose weight. Being disabled in some parts of your body is not enough to deter you from performing exercises. Everybody, however can eat less.

There are some athletes who have been physically-impaired but their minds made them stand fast towards their goal of keeping themselves fit in spite of their incapacity to perform other jobs. If this feat will merit your attention, then, there is no reason for you to hold on to that binding rope.

Pursuing the Goal
What do people usually do when they want to pursue a goal? They should have a drive and the right amount of motivation to freely transform their dream into a reality. Nevertheless, there must be a certain amount of planning; otherwise, nothing can be achieved and all of the efforts would be put to waste. Here are some of the ways that can help you obtain yours:

Be realistic: There is no such thing as a perfect workout and no perfect diet meal can be called successful unless your feet are still touching the ground. You have to know that success can come after a sacrifice and sacrifices involve risks that you have to take. Setting up a goal to achieve a desired weight does not give you results. It is the way you can reach it that can give you solutions to your everlasting dilemma. Therefore, never set a very high goal that you know is impossible for you to achieve.

Plan thoroughly: Planning takes time so you have to take one step at a time. It is said that sure answers are carefully thought of and being hasty brings you nowhere. Being impulsive can lead you to a path full of blunders so you better take note of what you have written on your priority list and act on it wisely.

Know your strengths: If you know where you are good at, then, you must practice it the way you control your cravings for food. Foods that can offer you too much cholesterol and fats may be avoided by some but to other dieters who are seeking to trim down on weight—it is impossible.
Asking for a nutritionist to aid you on your slimming program is best so you will have the right nutrients on your plate each time you take your meals.

Set a deadline: Deadlines work a lot for the improvement of one's weight loss program. Following your regimen to the dot can make you expect the right results at a time frame given to you by your fitness guru or your dietician.
No pain, no gain; that's what others say.

Ways to Keep your Goal Alive
There are many ways to keep your goal alive and this entails you to be very observant in a lot of aspects before and during fitness or diet programs. You may want to take a look at these:
- Look at your situation: Look at how your body has grown and try to figure out which among your body parts is giving you some embarrassment. Then, you may list down what you want to do with it. This is where you start planning on what measure to take to eliminate the unsightly area. My greatest problems

were my belly and my hips. They just would not fit into my old clothes. However, losing pounds by cutting down on what I ate also reduced my belly and my hips.

- Get some advice: Useful advice can be obtained from the masters or certified experts on health and fitness. These are the people you have to ask for help and not depend only on what your friends did to make them lose unwanted pounds.

- Follow instructions: Following a regimen to the last steps in a schedule provided by you or by your fitness instructor is a good idea. Set aside time for each activity or meal and be sure to do it regularly without cheating yourself.

- Be enthusiastic: Being enthusiastic on your diet and routines can give it more enjoyment than complaining about a small meal that makes you hungry every now and then; or a severe exercise phase that you don't really want to undergo. Make it more pleasant by pretending you like it and that you are out to get that desirable figure you have long pined for!

- Read more materials: There are testimonials that can motivate you into doing your program. You may read from the celebrities' testimonials or just from plain individuals that can boost your morale. These people have been through what you have experienced and their stories could serve to inspire you more.

- Be creative: If you think your diet meal doesn't go with your budget, you may ask your dietician for replacements. Learn how certain foods can be substituted by others that are available in your neighborhood and cheaper than those that can be ordered from other laces.

- Perform routines with a buddy: To create a more pleasant environment, you can invite a buddy who also needs to trim down so you can talk while on the gym. Lesser stress can be felt once you have somebody to talk to while performing your scheduled routines.

Chapter 3
Focusing on the Dieter

Many dieters often fail in their weight loss programs and there are different facets where we can look into these faults. Let us take the following types of dieters into consideration:

Dieter A is the type of person who looks forward to seeing great expectations. This person knows that there is a specific time frame set by fitness experts for each phase of the plan they are in; however, he wants to see results immediately. Is there a fast diet scheme? Of course, there is none because there are series of steps that one has to go about and a target goal for each phase included in the plan. Therefore, for a particular phase, there is a specific target that dieters have to obtain and that may give you access to the next goal.

Dieter B is the lazy individual. This person never follows a schedule and cheats every time he sees food. He is also capable of skipping an exercise routine whenever the fitness expert turns his head the other way. This is the one who has to be watched as even the most effective regimen would prove to be worthless or ineffective.

Dieter C is the cheapskate. Buying cheap to set aside money for the rainy days is a virtue but going cheap when choosing a fitness gym or instructor is a huge negative sign for this individual. This person may search for the cheapest gym in town that pays instructors at a minimal fee.

Now, gym participants may agree to be coached once in a blue moon by a so-called exercise expert who goes around the fitness center just to look at their patrons doing their own thing. Chances are the instructor is not even certified to offer a decent program to patrons as he might not have been trained for that!

Dieter D's focus is short term. Focusing on short-term goals is not a new thing for some individuals. These people's minds are set to get into an activity but after a while, there is a tendency to stop. Once they cannot seem to go beyond a scheduled phase of a certain program, they would back out as a result of frustration. This behavior goes beyond stopping as there would never be enough drive to make them continue doing their tasks.

Exercise can be really tough but once there is a will to overpower laziness or loss of drive, results are greater. It is not only in their new form that dieters would find satisfaction from but based on the effort that they have used, they would find it more gratifying to have taught themselves how to stick on to what they do and their achievement was done mainly because of their changed attitude towards things.

Always remember that not all advice coming from friends are good to hear; more so, if you are planning to embark on a weight loss program. Some may see it as a ploy so you can strike up an argument within the group. Others may look at it in a different way like getting attention as you have been missing in action recently. They might consider that you are already trying to evade them for reasons other than a weight loss goal.

You may hear unpleasant remarks that can make you lose your drive in the process. Somehow, there would be a few who would think that you are really bent on going through the ordeal if you are the type who complains about frequent nights out and spending irreverently as staying inside the house is your idea of relaxation. Don't forget that your friends have different opinions from what you have so expect the unexpected and try not to get swayed by anything.

If you really want to hear the best advice, contact a professional who can help you to face your fears before starting at anything. These are learned people who are experienced to deal with the things you want to undergo and authorities when it comes to handling behavior that goes with the dieter himself. Seasoned professionals could help you pass the first stage which is coping with being overweight that dieters always fail. Unless you feel the need to throw out the negativity in you, you might never succeed in this endeavor.

At the onset of the plan, think about building up confidence. If there is still some amount left in you, fuel it up by talking to family members. They can give you the hardest push. These are people who deeply care about you and the last thing they want to see in you is to become frustrated on how you look. Close family ties are made out of blood relations and bonding. Make love and understanding your essential gear in making your dream a reality. And maybe, there is truth when you say: *"where friends fail, family can help you make things work."*

Among the most common blunders that dieters would encounter is their inability to know the size or amount that they are allowed to take each meal. Portion or size matters and so as the weight of each ingredient that a nutritionist or dietitian has specified. With a restricted diet, one can surely be on his way towards the goal and doing assigned exercises can make it more effective.

If your nutritionist asks you to put in a particular ingredient and it stipulates a certain amount of weight or measurement, follow it to the dot. This will not hurt you a bit. Only your expanded stomach will complain about the process as it got used to large amounts of foods stashed on it for a certain period of time.

The habit of eating too much can be curbed by teaching yourself to go slow on food. Eating is an activity that the body needs and it brings forth nourishment to the body. Nevertheless, too much quantity leads to serious illnesses and a ticket towards obesity can be obtained by you for free!

Look into your diet plan. If you can see the phrase *'recommended serving'*, then, that is your cue. All sizes have a corresponding calorie and nutrient intake. Other than the suggested size will hamper the efficiency of the program. You may also be tempted to use alternative ingredients but be sure that to lessen the amount of sugar that has been required of the mixture. Fruits contain sugar so, in excess of a portion will not be good and may slow down the progress you want to see.

Never be like other shoppers who are not at all troubled by the same predicament such as yours. They'd buy food randomly just because they are fit. It is imperative that you look into the labels of each canned goods you buy or outside every package of the food on the gondolas of a supermarket. They contain nutrition facts and these are what you need to see. Never be blinded of the foods that you used to buy for dinner. You can just imagine that all because you did not have the time to cook healthy meals, you have amassed a good number of pounds which you have acquired from eating from fast-food chains or canned goods. But do not be obsessed to that and become a *can reader.*

Lifestyle Checking is best

Have you had any lifestyle checking lately? You might have forgotten that you need not live in abundance but just in moderation of almost anything that you have and want. We understand that what you want in life is what you are striving so hard for. This must be the reason why you have been working day in and day out. The standard of living we have is what makes us in the eyes of people who surround us. Nonetheless, our effort to afford what we desire boils down to one thing—lifestyle.

The kind of life we lead can be something that we can take pride on. On the other hand, the good life can also mean overindulgence to different sorts of things like food, alcohol and cigarettes. Cigarettes may lead us to cancer and other upper respiratory tract illnesses while eating in excess leads to obesity. Too much liquor is likewise addictive as it can transform a frequent drinker into an alcoholic.

Why are we tackling this topic when are talking about weight loss? It is in citing these examples that can bring some of us to our senses. People see us from a perspective and it is a fact that when a person has an addiction, he has the propensity to deny an observer's perception. Thus, people who overindulge on any activity do not even know they are deep into it. Regret comes when illness strikes. It is only then he'd come to realize the excesses in life that he has had splurged on.

Acceptance is the best way to clear away the cobwebs from our minds as we ponder on getting help for our problems. There can never be any solution if the mind is not willing to undergo change. Change comes from within and this voluntary action and submission gives way to a better life ahead. For as long as you lead a life of moderation, nothing can stand as your adversary but the number of years that you have spent in this world.

Wrong Foods and Wrong Exercise
Are you eating more than enough or just eat whenever you are hungry? This is a common question we throw to people who are either overweight or underweight for their age and body build. Underweight people think that they have eaten enough but the real thing is they do not eat what is right. If nutrients that enter our bodies are less than the required amount we have to take, then, it can be harmful to our health. It is vital that we follow the exact dose our body needs to consume to make us healthy inside and out. Even overweight people can be considered as undernourished because they are not eating right as well.

What they tend to eat are only foods they want to swallow. This notion is wrong as there should be a balanced diet for every one of us in order to stay longer. So, when they become heavier, they would enroll in weight training classes or go on a crash diet, which is also not advised according to health experts. Crash dieting has a lot of consequences. It may take us to undergo rigid exercise routines that could kill, and leaves us to abstain from eating for days.

We sometimes fail on our aim to lessen our food intake right after we have seen how much we weigh at a certain point of time. This signals the crash diet tendency or we think that it is the number one solution for our failure to control our urge to eat. Some persons think that crash dieting is the key to weigh loss once again as they only take in minimal amounts of food. It is actually an unreasonable scheme that we should avoid. Crash diets can take on different types of meal plans but uses only a fraction of the basic food groups that the body need to consume daily.

Now, if there is a crash scheme for meals, it also has a counterpart in the world of exercise. For the simple reason that there is a need to eliminate fats from the body, other people who are knowledgeable of how a wrong exercise scheme can hurt the entire body would ask for the fastest remedy. Some enterprising fitness centers would promise to deliver your dream body in weeks. Don't fret; many people have asked for this type of cure and may even have included one of your friends. There is no such thing as the fastest cure; only perseverance can help you in your endeavor.

Chapter 4
Weight Loss Program Issues

Never let stress bother you even if you have grown so big that you think a weighing scale would complain every time you step on it. Life doesn't end there, friend. There's more to what life can offer than just sulking because you have grown bigger—and heavier. You can change that by means of arming yourself with great determination to succeed on your weight loss plan.

Stress is just around the corner and it devours an individual who cannot handle it well. There is something called stress management and you can use that against the word itself and the battle can be won once you know where to start. Stress is a product of being overly involved with a particular issue and an issue like being overweight can take a toll on some individual's life and health. Being into this situation can be very daunting as the person who is undergoing stress may not be able to cope with it alone. It is advisable to seek professional help or advice in order to take away this negative feeling.

Weighing above normal is an issue to some people but others don't even care about it. There are individuals who take pride on how they look and seem to be happy about it; and this goes for both fat and thin people. Persons who are too stressed out with their appearance may succumb to becoming heavier as they would tend to eat more without noticing it.

After that, they would find out that they have grown wider on the hips, and not a lean part of their body can be seen by the naked eye.

Right immediately after a consultation with a physician who may direct you to a nutritionist, exercise regimen follows. However, there is still the troubled mind to think about and this is what is to be dealt with. The person must bear in mind that the cure must emanate from within and that no medication can actually take it off unless the mind is willing to forego the feeling. The best remedy is to start treating yourself with a dose of happiness; think of happy thoughts to arrive at a different stage in your psyche. It is then you will find yourself treading the path towards fulfilling your goal which is to lose those extra pounds you might have helped amassed.

Being meticulous is good most importantly when the thing you're dealing with is shaving those pounds off your body. It is vital for every dieter to be very particular with details that even the smallest of them must be thoroughly checked. True to every fitness experts and health professionals, calorie counting, weight measurement, and time consumed during exercise must be recorded to see how the body that performs it reacts to a particular program.

Fitness trainers look forward to a day with their clients at the gym and with this in mind, they also get excited once they see progress on their wards. It is not only in the payments that they are looking forward to see at every scheduled date; they are more enthused about the positive changes in the bodily appearance of the person who go there to trim down. That is where their satisfaction from work is gained. That is why it pays to be meticulous in providing details to the dieters. If one move fails, the rest follows.

Dieticians already know how many calories are found on almost any food. They are persons who are more knowledgeable on this aspect when it comes to counting the calories and nutrients that go inside our body in the form of food. So, it makes sense when we say that any body type with a specific height measurement can only take in a specific number of calories daily if the aim is to lose some weight.

Weight has to be monitored every time a dieter checks in for a round of fitness routine. Weight checking is crucial for you to know and for the instructor to see so they will see if the program is working or not. They would begin to ask themselves once there is no positive change on the weight of a coached individual. This goes to show that the plan is not working. What they would do next is to check on the program itself to find out what seemed to have gone wrong.

A deadline is set in every program offered to each client inside a gym or even at home. This is where you will find yourself beating a certain date to get the results you want. Time frames in performing exercises are patterned to your diet and your lifestyle to make it work. Without a deadline, there are no specific results to watch out for.

Procrastination is a Bully
Why do some people refer to procrastination as a bully? It is because while a person is striving hard to get through his goal, he would pass at a stage wherein he deviates from the normal and clear path towards the realization of his dreams. In such case, the drive stops; thus, the final thrust of a project never materializes.

This is also true when it comes to losing weight. People, no matter how they try and spend for a weight loss program, may or may not accomplish it due to some reasons they alone know. But this behavior can be overturned once it begins to show up on your system by means of concentrating on your determination to succeed.

Focus your mind and think of the benefits of getting a leaner form. This will make you feel at ease and the better for you to gear up for the next round of routines your instructor has prepared for you.

Here are a few examples on why there is a stoppage of task performance:

Budget constraints: Somewhere along the way, a dieter stops from doing his chores because of lack of funds to continue on. But things may be different if one begins a program with an amount of savings that can help him push through with his goal.

Lack of energy: A person who longs to shed off pounds may stop for the reason that he got exhausted with the rigid exercise routines that were assigned to him. It is essential, therefore, to ask a reliable trainer to offer you with routines that would not burn out the person performing them. Overdoing a program may lead to exhaustion and this may be the case of a lot of people who have the same aim.

Mid-project disappointment: Never hasten up the results of the program you are in. There is no other way to get pleasant results than taking it slow but surely, and thinking of a way to make routines more enjoyable and you can do this with friends. This way, you will never get tired with your regimen as you look forward to meet up with your buddies at a gym.

Testimonials can add up to the Motivation

What happens when you read testimonials from people who have been successful in battling obesity? It would seem like you want to try what they have experienced too, right? There is always a positive reaction upon reading how other people have become successful. Nevertheless, there are also some skeptics who would not even dare to test the waters not because they think of those measures as ineffective but they are not so sure if they can overcome the issue the same as the ones before them.

There would always be negative reactions upon reading testimonies coming from people who have tried different measures to battle the bulge. This is but natural as sometimes, testimonials can be edited and graphic results can be rigged to appear that particular weight loss measures are really effective. This is what advertising does to their target markets. But there are some of them that can offer really good results. Setting aside being skeptical, why not read reviews first in order to get an insight on the effectiveness of a particular program than become doubtful about what it can offer you?

Of course there is also a wrong thinking that weight loss measures that your friends haven't tried yet would fail. This is what we hear from a dieter who is not bent on proceeding to take off the excess weight he owns. The person would try to read testimonies from previously fat people, laugh at what they say, and would not even do a thing to seek a better advice for his own welfare.

If you have read testimonials and have been amazed at their results, you may assign yourself to use them as a guide in doing things that can make you shed those unwanted weight. To be sure, you may ask fitness or medical professionals if the measures are good for you. Your health condition has to be considered so as to make it work for your own well-being.

Getting into a weight loss program may be a very hard thing for you to sustain. First, you have to put up with the time you need to perform the program alone, as it involves a fraction of your waking hours. Next, you must be contented with meals that are quite different from what you have indulged in for quite a time. If these seem to bother you a lot, then, weight loss issues will be yours forever unless you start doing something to make the problem go away.

Here are some tips that you may use for your goal but not necessarily to use them altogether.

- *Never watch TV while eating* - Watching your favorite sitcom or TV series can make you eat more. As you watch the show, you will tend to forget that you can only eat so much.

- *Delete snack time forever* - Taking in food in between meals can add up to your weight and calorie intake. Even if you say that you have just chewed a burger, think of the calories that it can give you. If you cannot delete the snack completely, grab a very small bag of chips and try not to finish it alone by sharing it with someone.

- *Exercise at least three times in a week* – Never forget to do some crunches to sculpt your body's landscape. This will give you results that you can be proud of. A little crunching goes a long, long way.

- *Forget about bar-hopping* – Liquor, no matter how small the amount, once added up may give you several liters of booze inside your system. As we already know, liquor can make your belly grow and as you take a sip, you also take some finger foods on the side.

- *Full breakfast meals are best* – Eating a good, not heavy breakfast with protein and carbs can surely balance blood sugar levels. This also makes you forget to eat a hearty lunch.

- *Linger on the bed* – Take time to stay on the bed several minutes than you used to before and after sleep. This may give you clearer options on the best meal that can help you lose weight.

- *Fruits can be your best friends* – Eating a couple of fruits in the morning or within the day gives in to a healthy digestive system and good skin. However, this can also make you feel full and cravings for food become lesser in volume. Someone has suggested eating an apple each time before your meal so that the apple fills up the space you would have otherwise filled with calories you don't need.

- *Never forget to monitor your weight* – Of all the things that you do, be sure to monitor your weight by tipping the scale every day. This way, you will be able to see where your program is going; whether you are falling off form the normal weight or going overboard by having eaten a lot at a party.

Chapter 5
Action Plan

There are some factors that you must consider before you can create an action plan that would serve as your weight loss inspiration. You have to know what it stands for and you must know if it would really work for you. But how can you determine if the plan would actually work to gain results? Let us find answers to this question.

Action plans are drafted schedules of activities to do and may tell you what to avoid before going about a certain program. They are sets of guidelines to follow in order to achieve success. Some creators of action plans may give you options while others may draft severe technique-laden ones to ensure accomplishment of a project.

Top factors included in an action plan:
- *Goal* – The core is the goal with which the doer pictures out as the target and a means of motivation like a dog to a bone.

- *Time frame or deadline* – No task is definite and results may not be complete if there is no respect for the time scheduled for it to materialize.

- *Strategies* – Plans can be drafted with either simple tasks or complex ones but the common denominator would always be the time specified by the drafter.

Things may work out well by using an action plan which is necessary for the improvement of a person's physical appearance like weight loss programs. There can never be any good outcome if the program that was crafted for a participant is not accomplished to the last step. Following a plan that was made for a specific individual may just work for anyone else. Full motivation can be sustained when the person who is into the routine follows it religiously.

Here are some steps you have to take when aiming to pursue your dream of becoming leaner and fit and making your action plan effective:

Know what you want to achieve. Before anything else, know what you want to obtain and make it simple. Frustration is just in the corner; so, never allow it to set in. You can dream big but keep it to a level.

Make sure you reach some milestones on the way. Once you set your eyes on a target, you have to be ready for the milestones. Recognize something that you have achieved and write it down. This may not only fuel up your drive but will serve to add to the enthusiasm to accomplish the goal.

Break down larger targets into smaller ones. If in case a target is not achieved easily, you can break it down into smaller bits to make it more obtainable

Create a deadline for every target. Each time you are into a program, make sure you get it done on a schedule as specified at the onset.

Sustain your motivation. Keep the flame alive by means of further motivating yourself. You may use some inspiration along the way like a friend's successful weight loss program's tale or a celebrity's successful trek into becoming slim again.

Rearrange but don't give up. If everything fails, get back to it and try a different approach. Hold on to your dream of taking off those undesirable fats and feel like you're on top of the world.

You can draft your own plan according to how you picture out your results and use them by taking slow or small steps that are sure enough to propel you to reach your goal.

- *Never hasten the process* - Not all things can be sped up just to finish it. There is nothing you can do to hasten up a program that was made to be done and patterned to last a particular time frame. Blunders abound in the road towards slim individuals so don't be on a rush to get there.

- *Stay calm while on the program* - Controlling the hype while on a program gives you a more relaxed persona and relaxed muscles. Being peaceful in your adventurous travel to the slimming world prevents cramped muscles and a stressful mind.

- *Get on your feet and do the tasks* - Always be reminded that you have an obligation towards yourself once you have agreed to join a weight trimming program. Sleep is a luxury but never go out without it. One thing more— be enthusiastic about your routine as this can give you more enjoyment rather than complaints.

- *Build up confidence* - Confidence is slowly built even while you are still in the middle of the program. This means that you believe in yourself and you know that you can finish the tasks appointed to you by your trainer.

- *Focus on a reward* - Focus on something that you can award yourself after your program has ended. Every program is deemed to end; so, you have to think of an item which you have long sought after to serve as a gift for endurance and patience.

If there are so many things to think about like paying for a trainer and buying foods that would comprise your diet meal, you can always work it out within yourself. You can be creative sometimes so that you may save some money on the side. Listed below are some money-saving tips you can use upon having decided to get on with your weight loss program.

- *Your fitness expert* - Consult friends regarding a trainer that charges not so much but can guarantees results. Since there are fitness experts inside a fitness center, there may be some who can work during off duty or at times when they are not busy with other jobs. These people may offer you a lower charging fee.

- *Deciding to start* – You had better decided once and for all when to start on a program and be sure not to turn back. Indecision means spending more on your part; so, do away with this trend of thought. You can always choose your own schedule so better be honest in telling your trainer about your times available.

- *Scheduling woes* – If you are into a certain fitness program, be sure that you can arrive on time so as not to go hasty in doing the routines. Skipping one session makes you lose many opportunities. Scheduled time frames are deemed to be followed, thus, you have to ensure that you are on the right track and right on schedule.

- *Food supplements* – You may or may not use these as to supplement your diet meals as they are not that essential. As long as you eat a balanced diet and a healthy breakfast, you should be able to finish your program on time.

Ways to Reach your Desired Weight
If there are various ways to create an action plan, there are different ways that can help you achieve your desired weight as well. We have just listed two of the most common measures that serve as your guide.

1. Calculate the number of calorie intake

Burning calories everyday also needs you to replenish them by eating a good number of calories in a day which is approximately 1200 for female weight loss participants and for the males—that would be 1500 calories. Therefore, calories burned must be over the number of calorie intake. Never be overhyped with your program that you tend to overdo on the routines while cutting back a little bit of your food intake. This may lead you to a deficit that may endanger your health.

Burning 2 pounds every week is not bad. The body needs to adjust to the lesser intake so, keep it that way to obtain better results. You may also look at the type of activity you are into as this may need you to add some amount of food to fuel you up if your regimen is rigid.

2. Assessing your ideal weight

You can learn to assess your weight by means of the Body Mass Index or BMI formula which is based on your weight and height. This determines if you are at risk or not. Factors that are involved are age and build. Working out a BMI at a range of 18.5-24.9 is normal. That means:
Weight in kilograms ÷ Height (m) x height or kg ÷ mx2 = BMI
This measurement was designed for both males and females with ages ranging from 18-65 years old. A better understanding on how to measure your BMI may be a good thing for those who seek to trim down on undesirable body mass.

Chapter 6

Choosing the Right Program for you

Of all the diet programs you have seen, which among them do you think is good for you?

Did you know that there is an appropriate diet plan for each and every one of us? We simply cannot go on a diet for the reason that we have to get some mass from our body. There has to be proper consultation with a physician or a diet expert before starting it out on the road towards a healthy way of life.

Things to consider are: your goal, preferences, your medical history and your budget. These three things are essential to know because it is in these aspects that the success of your endeavor depends on. Let's take each of the aspects one by one.

Your goal is what propels you to do an activity. So, if the activity involved is planning for weight loss, then, list your expectations but keep them on a reasonable level. Never go for a goal that you are not able to keep up. Your goals will be edited by your dietitian once he or she sees it. That is one of the merits of having someone who is an authority in the field.

 Your preferences may not be among those of health experts. For one, you will be listing the food you would want to see on your plate while he lists what you are to eat at a particular time and day.

So, say goodbye to too much carbohydrates and fats; say hello to a stricter meal that would not kill you in the process but may give you a better health and figure.

If you opt to go on a diet alone, think about the type of person you are. If you have cheated on your diet in the past, then, you are more likely to cheat on it again. You can also go with a group who can share their experiences with you. There are online diet groups that you can join. If you want to get an audience, then, let it be a respected family member. This will enable you to tread on the right path.

Your medical history counts as an ideal gauge. Having an erratic blood pressure disallows you to eat some of the ingredients of a diet plan. This record has to be checked by your health specialist so that person can give appropriate consideration. There are alternatives to what you want to avoid.

Budget has to be checked as well as given consideration. Be sure that you know where to purchase cheaper ingredients. You must be able to know how to keep them fresh so by the time you want to cook them, they are not stale.

If there are other things that you want to be considered, you may talk it out with your food specialist as he knows what to say and knows what would work for you best.

Best Fitness Venue in the Eyes of a Beginner

If you are new to weight loss programs, then, you have to know the type of exercises that are involved or appropriate for you. To start with, prepare yourself for the worst. Not all exercise routines are easy. If at the start you are given something that requires maximum movement, don't smile or get bored.

It is just a beginning of a long road ahead. It is unavoidable for a beginner to think this way as they think that regimens offered by fitness gurus are supposedly tense and nerve-wrecking.

In the eyes of a beginner, fitness venues should be complete with all the facilities and the instructors are there whenever they need them. Trainers are not that many in other venues. An exercise location does not hire one trainer each for every patron that enrolls in a program. Proper scheduling are what they do best so that every time a client comes in and asks for his or her routine, everything is ready and there is someone to assist them in a particular duration.

Certified training experts are those whom you see as systematic in performing their duties. They have instilled a sense of responsibility towards people who hire them for the task. Once they are consulted, they would see to it that the list of exercises is right for the person who will perform it. Thus, there has to be complete understanding on the type of trainee they have; otherwise, these people would suffer from miscalculation of capabilities and medical condition could worsen.

Beginners lean towards perfection and too much expectation. Again, expectations on this type of patrons must be curbed so they will not suffer from frustration. They might be disgruntled by the way they were handled as they have expected too much. Some of them may leave the program and never to come back again.

As the routines get harder, the trainer is tasked to warn the newbies on how the next phase is performed and explain how they would be able to take the rigors of the training. Interacting with a weight loss participant is a good measure.

This alleviates them from the hard regimen they are into and the next ones they have to undergo.

How to sustain your goal is what you have to aim for. There are many things that you can do in order for you to continue and reach your target on the right schedule. The first step is to learn to do what you are tasked to do. Never think of it as a task but a regimen that can deliver utmost satisfaction. Diets and exercises can be fun for people of all ages who are willing to forego their bellies and sagging arms; not to mention cellulite that has used their thighs as habitat! If this is you, don't feel offended, but let this propel you to action. You may ask for some varieties from your trainer who has a lot in store for you. Your willingness to do routines will furthermore propel you to go with it until everything is done.

Exercising with a group or your best friend may be a suggestion that you wouldn't want to say no to. It would be more fun doing crunches with people who are also into your kind of thing. Exchanging experiences and feelings while on a plan is almost the same as exchanging pleasantries. This lessens the burden of assigned routines; next thing you know, you are done for the day!

Use music to lessen the stress while working out. This may distract you a bit but getting used to it is what you should do. You will never count the minutes that you have been training once there is music on your ears. So, prepare your headset and save music that ranges from slow to medium to fast.

Breathing can be done with the music. Find something that fits the pace of your routine. When at home, dance to the beat of rock whenever you can find time. It can be while you are cooking or wiping the furniture.

Never forget to stretch before and after your workout. It won't hurt if you do but definitely hurts the entire body if you don't. Lastly, always bring a bottle of water to replenish what you have perspired. Water never adds to your weight!

Losing weight is not only dependent on the meals and exercises that were assigned to the dieter. The kind of food that is involved in each meal plan must be carefully thought out and prepared according to the plan. Your nutritionist may have an idea on how these foods are cooked or prepared so you have to take note to the last detail. If some ingredients are to be served and eaten raw, they have to be raw; if the meal states that the fish has to be cooked in olive oil, then, so be it.

Another thing that must be watched out is the kind of food that goes in certain food groups. It is essential to know this as your meals have to contain all food groups every time they are served. So, if fish does not come in handy at your nearby grocery, then, beef may take its place. It is to be noted that fiber can be derived not only from vegetables and fruits; they can also be obtained from fish and meat. On the other hand, instead of getting fats from a slice of pork, you can get some from nuts.

Knowing how to get a balanced diet is quite important for a dieter and much more needed by beginners. Where do you get a list of the food groups? Learning more means reading more. Make it a point to ask questions from the proper authority so you can be enlightened by things that stands as your blind spot.

If everything else fails, you may connect with friends. They may know something that you don't. These people, have, in one way or another, been through the same predicament so bond with them or never forget to tap their help when the need arises.

Seeking Professional Advice from Experts
Being aware of different kinds of exercise and diet plans may be a good proposition as opting for programs that don't go with the dieter's schedule and body capabilities may aggravate the situation. This is where weight loss programs prove to be ineffective towards the user and the most common problem that could make them back out.

Exercise programs can be tough and some of them may be too lenient for an individual dieter. Always remember that each person is unique and that exercise must be patterned on the type of body each one has. There is also much consideration to be given to the health conditions of every dieter involved. You may not be able to use the rigid program that the others are using, thus, getting some medical advice from your physician is best.

Listen to what the trainer or dietitian has to say. Motivating words can either calm you down or push you more to the targets that were set. Try not to deviate from your course to ensure the success of your program. Or better yet, maintain your pace at a certain speed as hurrying out to the end is not the answer to your problem.
Professionals who work to help provide you with a better well-being are supposedly dedicated so there's no need for you to panic. Loss of confidence on the experts is the result of panic; so, you have to try your best to eradicate this feeling out of your system. Using an open-mind towards what is laid in front of you gives you more possibilities of succeeding.

Principles of safe food handling:
1. Personal hygiene of the food handler
   - Wash hands thoroughly with soap and water before handling food.
   - Use clean utensils for taste testing.
   - Avoid preparing food when sick.

2. Kitchen sanitation
   - Clean surfaces and dishes with hot water and detergent
   - Cutting boards – Plastic is preferable to wood for cleaning
   - Prepare raw foods separately from meats to be cooked
   - Thoroughly wash and scrub fresh fruits and vegetables before serving.

3. Storage conditions and practices
   - Food temperatures maintained below 40° or above 140°
   - Avoid storing protein-containing foods at room temperature over 2 hours
   - Keep meats in the lowest part of the refrigerator to avoid contamination
   - Keep storage areas clean to avoid contamination of new foods
   - Store foods properly as soon as possible after purchase
   - Buy only quantities you will use before spoilage can occur

Basic Food Categories

What are the different Categories?
- ❖ **Carbohydrate**
- ❖ **Fiber**
- ❖ **Fat**
- ❖ **Protein**

Carbohydrates:
- Compounds composed of single or multiple sugars.
- Complex carbohydrates are long chains of sugars.
- Glucose from carbohydrates is the preferred fuel for the body.
- In general should comprise 55-60% of the diet.

Fiber:
- Composed of long chains of sugars that humans cannot digest.
- Classified as soluble and insoluble based on how they dissolve in water.
- Benefits of fiber: promotes fullness, prevents constipation, prevents diverticulosis, reduces the risk for colon cancer, heart and artery disease, improves glucose control and may help lower blood cholesterol.

Fat:
- Triglyceride is one of the main classes of dietary lipids.
- Essential fatty acids are fats the body needs but cannot make. Omega-6 fatty acids are essential. They are found in vegetable oils, seeds, nuts, and whole grains. Omega-3 fatty acids are also essential and are found

primarily in fatty fish and to a lesser degree in flax seed and canola oil.

- Saturated fatty acids/Monounsaturated fatty acids/Polyunsaturated fatty acids differ in the number and point of saturation. This affects the hardness of the fat at room temperature and has differing effects on blood lipids and heart disease risk.
- Trans fats are produced through hydrogenation. Trans fats elevate bad LDL cholesterol and lower beneficial HDL. This may lead to even greater heart disease risk than saturated fats.
- In general fat should be limited to 20-30% of the diet.

Protein:

- Distinctive because they contain nitrogen and are made up of amino acids. There are nine essential amino acids that must be supplied by the diet.
- Supports numerous bodily functions:
  - o Protein supports growth and maintenance in the body – building new tissue and replacing worn-out cells.
  - o Enzymes, hormones, and other chemicals are formed from proteins.
  - o Proteins build antibodies to defend against foreign proteins.
  - o They are critical for maintaining fluid and electrolyte balance.
  - o Acid-base balance, blood ph, is maintained by protein's buffering capacity.
  - o Proteins transport substances such as lipids, minerals and oxygen in the body.
  - o Emergency energy to fuel body functions can also be produced from proteins.

- Protein quality is determined by its amino acids, digestibility and how well it supports growth.
- Complete proteins are found in meat, dairy, eggs, and soy products. Incomplete proteins are found in grains, legumes, nuts and seeds. When eaten in combination the proteins are complementary and meet amino acid needs.

In general, most people need approximately 0.8 g protein per kg body weight. 15-20% of the diet should be high quality protein

Low Fat/ Low Cholesterol Diet

A low fat/ low cholesterol diet, along with exercise and medications, is useful in improving blood cholesterol levels. There are many types of cholesterol. The total cholesterol and low-density lipoprotein ("bad cholesterol") should be kept as low as possible. The high-density lipoprotein ("good cholesterol") is best to keep as high as possible.

The body needs cholesterol for several important functions. It makes blood cholesterol from the fat and cholesterol in the diet. Since the body makes all the cholesterol it needs, it is not necessary to eat cholesterol-containing foods. Cholesterol is only found in foods of animal origin, including meat, fish, shellfish, eggs and dairy products.

Breads, cereals, rice and pasta

> Choose whole-grain or enriched breads,
> cereals, rice and pasta. Choose low-fat and
> fat-free crackers. Avoid breads prepared
> with eggs or cheese, granola, biscuits,
> muffins, pancakes and pastries.

Fruits and vegetables

All fresh, frozen, canned and dried fruits and vegetables are
recommended.
Avoid vegetables prepared with fat, cream sauce or cheese
sauce.

Milk, Yogurt and Cheese

Choose skim, nonfat and fat-free milk, cheese and yogurt.
Avoid 2% milk, whole milk, cream and regular cheese.
Substitute evaporated skim milk for whole milk and cream.

Meats, poultry, fish, dry beans, eggs and nuts

Lean cuts of meat, skinless poultry and fish packed in water
are recommended. Choose legumes cooked without fat.
Avoid fatty cuts of meat, most luncheon meats and egg
yolks.

Basics for Handling Food Safely

Safe steps in food handling, cooking, and storage are essential to prevent foodborne illness. You can't see, smell, or taste harmful bacteria that may cause illness. In every step of food preparation, follow the four Fight BAC!™ guidelines to keep food safe:

- Clean — Wash hands and surfaces often.
- Separate — Don't cross-contaminate.
- Cook — Cook to proper temperatures.
- Chill — Refrigerate promptly.

Shopping

- Purchase refrigerated or frozen items after selecting your non-perishables.
- Never choose meat or poultry in packaging that is torn or leaking.
- Do not buy food past "Sell-By," "Use-By," or other expiration dates.

Storage

- Always refrigerate perishable food within 2 hours (1 hour when the temperature is above 90 °F).
- Check the temperature of your refrigerator and freezer with an appliance thermometer. The refrigerator should be at 40 °F or below and the freezer at 0 °F or below.
- Cook or freeze fresh poultry, fish, ground meats, and variety meats within 2 days; other beef, veal, lamb, or pork, within 3 to 5 days.

- Perishable food such as meat and poultry should be wrapped securely to maintain quality and to prevent meat juices from getting onto other food.
- To maintain quality when freezing meat and poultry in its original package, wrap the package again with foil or plastic wrap that is recommended for the freezer.
- In general, high-acid canned food such as tomatoes, grapefruit, and pineapple can be stored on the shelf for 12 to 18 months. Low-acid canned food such as meat, poultry, fish, and most vegetables will keep 2 to 5 years — if the can remains in good condition and has been stored in a cool, clean, and dry place. Discard cans that are dented, leaking, bulging, or rusted.

Preparation

- Always wash hands before and after handling food.
- Don't cross-contaminate. Keep raw meat, poultry, fish, and their juices away from other food. After cutting raw meats, wash hands, cutting board, knife, and counter tops with hot, soapy water.
- Marinate meat and poultry in a covered dish in the refrigerator.
- Sanitize cutting boards by using a solution of 1 teaspoon chlorine bleach in 1 quart of water.

Thawing

- **Refrigerator**: The refrigerator allows slow, safe thawing. Make sure thawing meat and poultry juices do not drip onto other food.
- **Cold Water**: For faster thawing, place food in a leak-proof plastic bag. Submerge in cold tap water. Change the water every 30 minutes. Cook immediately after thawing.
- **Microwave**: Cook meat and poultry immediately after microwave thawing.

Cooking

- Beef, veal, and lamb steaks, roasts, and chops may be cooked to 145 °F.
- All cuts of pork, 160 °F.
- Ground beef, veal and lamb to 160 °F.
- All poultry should reach a safe minimum internal temperature of 165 °F.

Serving

- Hot food should be held at 140 °F or warmer.
- Cold food should be held at 40 °F or colder.
- When serving food at a buffet, keep food hot with chafing dishes, slow cookers, and warming trays. Keep food cold by nesting dishes in bowls of ice or use small serving trays and replace them often.
- Perishable food should not be left out more than 2 hours at room temperature (1 hour when the temperature is above 90 °F).

Leftovers

- Discard any food left out at room temperature for more than 2 hours (1 hour if the temperature was above 90 °F).
- Place food into shallow containers and immediately put in the refrigerator or freezer for rapid cooling.
- Use cooked leftovers within 4 days.

Refreezing
Meat and poultry defrosted in the refrigerator may be refrozen before or after cooking. If thawed by other methods, cook before refreezing.

Food Safety and Inspection Service. (2006). *Fact Sheets Safe Food Handling.*

http://www.fsis.usda.gov/Fact_Sheets/Basics_for_Handling _Food_Safely/index.asp.
Washington DC: United States Department of Agriculture.

Chapter 7
The Gym and the Experts

Before embarking on a fitness program, all you need is to get some pieces of advice from an able professional However, if you are in a dilemma when choosing who the best person for the job is, then, you may be interested in finding out what the listed professionals below can do:

Physicians
In your effort to lose weight, you may first approach your family physician as he would know best about your medical condition and the amount of fats that you need to shed off to get into a normal weight. Lest you have forgotten that you are into some kind of illness, your physician would know if you are prepared to tackle some rigid routines to get on to your goal.

Personal trainers
Personal trainers or fitness gurus are the people that you can find at fitness gyms. They are experts in body sculpting and exercise. However, these people would still like to see your medical history coming from your physician so they will know that you are deemed fit by a medical professional to undergo training. Experienced trainers require you to submit a doctor's physical examination before drafting a program for you.

Dietitian or nutritionist

Any of these two experts on food and nutrition can help you with your diet meal programs. They have learned what the body needs and know how to control food intake by creating an appropriate diet program for individuals. They can explain to you the meaning of BMI and can calculate your body mass by means of a formula. These individuals can work hand in hand with a personal trainer. And alongside your medical records, your program may become a successful one once you get a good advice from any of these two professionals.

Assessing a fitness gym that you can register in for the purpose of losing weight is easy once you know what you are expecting to get. There are just a few factors that need to be considered so you can start on your program right away.

Be sure that your chosen venue is easy highly accessible. Base its location on the distance that you have to travel from your home or from your workplace. It is imperative that you arrive on time before your fitness regimen starts to enable you to rest a little and adjust your body temperature to the environment.

Fitness venues do not charge the same. Some that charges lower than the others may not have complete facilities. You have to be sure that what your instructor requires you to undertake can be catered by the place that you have selected; otherwise, your effort will be put to waste. It pays to enroll in a center that has everything you need. Start asking questions on packages that they offer. You can be lucky to find a promo for your first month. That's already a clear savings on your part.

Get the best by asking around or browsing from the Internet. Gyms may advertise and brag that they have this and that in their facility but in fact, once you conduct an ocular inspection, they would lack some of what you need. Give it time to see if instructors are around. You can't just go into your routine alone. Personal assistance may be the best thing that a fitness center can offer their valued patrons.

Exercise is only a fraction of what we call weight loss program. The two other parts involve diet plan and the will of the mind to succeed. It is easy to spot the right fitness gym for you. However, it is harder to detect if the person whom you have commissioned as a personal trainer is really good unless you have heard it from the grapevine or have started and ended a program with the same individual.

Somehow, you can start from scratch by following the steps below:

1. Continuing education - An excellent fitness expert is one who doesn't stop learning. The professional in him gives him more room to learn new techniques and his work revolves around passion. Continual education is the key to added learning and this act benefits the clients who rely on their expertise.

2. Experience - Brilliant trainers are those who have worked for a long time in this kind of field. Expertise gained through experience is always the best thing that can happen to fitness experts. Everything goes on smoothly if the person you have commissioned for the task is well-versed with what

he does and with more learning comes integrity which is an essential part of the program.

3. Method of teaching - Sought-after fitness trainers have a way of making their clients understand the importance of each technique. They make sure clients understand the consequences if they do not perform well and may be glad to learn about the results if they do it right in due time. Motivating customers is something that they do best as well.

4. Understanding the client - Some clients may have a cloud over their heads and some of them are into depression; this is when the trainers come to think of ways to counter these predicaments. They know very well where their wards come from so, they give them assurance on what they can do and how they can alleviate the lifestyle of their patrons.

Exercising does not give you the right to eat more. This is one of the most famous blunders of people who are into weight loss plans. Several of them think that they can eat what they want as long as they are into a certain program. 'Let the program take care of me', as they say. However, no matter how they try to lose some pounds, they approach a dead end.

Exercise and eating always go together when into a diet program and there are no other excuses. One thing that one has to remember is that it's easy to lose weight only if you have a strong will to say no to something you think would exceed your quota for the day.

Keeping yourself away from possible weight-giving activities like eating can be your ticket towards a healthier lifestyle and a healthier-looking you. That means, if you work out to burn 300 calories or a pound of fat; avoiding an additional 300 calorie intake may give you twice as much the results you want. If you go through this the normal way, you may achieve only half the number in losing a pound. Imagine going through 12 sessions to lose 3,500 calories to weigh a pound lighter!

If people say they have slow metabolism, it doesn't follow that they burn calories slower than those who are active. It was proven that even while sitting down, calories are burned. What is true is slow eaters can consume more calories and can achieve a heavyweight status if they continue doing so within a week. It takes a lot of effort to eradicate the effects of drinking more than a couple of beers as well.

Exercise frequency is normal at three times a week with a little more than an hour's duration each. Given that you only consume 1,200 calories in a day, you can get ahead of the pack of exercisers inside the fitness venue you are at. Therefore, if you want to lose weight keep off from being lazy; get on your feet and hit the gym. Remind yourself not to overdo it, same as your food intake so you can arrive at the best results.

Losing weight cannot be done overnight. It's like moving a huge pile of rocks in a month or several months more; most especially if you are not following what your program dictates. This is the case of some people and this sometimes results to a very frustrating feeling. Depression which you want to take out comes in and out of the system as you unfalteringly fall short of things to get done with.

Expectations must be put to a normal level as the dilemma doesn't stop at losing pounds of unwanted body mass; disappointments over not having reached the goal can become an additional issue for the dieter. It is but natural to think of getting things done fast and easy but that is not how it works.

There's an equivalent date as scheduled by a trainer or a nutritionist before you may see the outcome of a particular program. Maybe, this is why some dieters back out from the activity by the time they cannot see results after a week or two.

Anticipating failure is a common feeling that fitness and diet meal patrons experience. This feeling is understood by each trainer or nutritionist. They know where these people are coming from; thus, there is a great need of making them understand the dos and don'ts of the trade and also ask them not to expect too much. Everything depends on the effort put up by their wards. So, if there is a leniency towards the program, results can also be minimal. Nevertheless, if the effort put up is huge, then, there is no way for them to fail.

The following is an excerpt from my book "Accept Challenges". I am including it in this book because you need to accept the challenge of the weight loss program.

Define the type of challenge you are dealing with and its elements

–Write out exactly what the components are that make up your challenge

–This allows you to plan ahead when setting goals, or to deal with things when they come up

–Anticipate what overcoming your challenge will involve

–Plan to overcome them in advance

Ways to overcome challenges

Plan, plan, plan

Be clear about your goals

Write them down

Be specific

Write out what challenges you expect will get in your way

Break them down into parts

Plan out how you deal with each part, and the challenge as a whole

Cultivate Awareness

Be aware of challenges when they occur

Be open to seeing them – don't keep your head in the sand

If you can't see it, you can't overcome it

You are keeping an eye out for opportunities

–To change

–To grow

–To get better

Once you have defined the challenge

Make a preliminary plan

Identify where the plan still needs work

Brainstorm solutions

Get help when needed
—Mentors/Coaches/Partners
—Counseling/Additional Employees/Teachers
Integrate solutions and advice from helpers into your plan

Path to success

Continually meeting challenges, overcoming them, and experiencing growth
Challenge→Overcome→Growth→Challenge (etc. circular info graphic)
It is a process
Challenges help us become who we are supposed to be
Embrace them
Don't be afraid
As when you were a child learning to crawl, walk, jump, play sports···.
Growth is good
It makes you better, stronger, smarter, more confident
Actively seek out challenges to become a better person
Continue to challenge yourself throughout your life
New skills and hobbies
Continual growth
Decide what you want to do, then go do it!
See challenges when they occur, and jump to overcome them
Challenges = Opportunity
Don't miss out

Things that spur us on
May be different for everyone
Figure out what works for you
Might be more than one

In Competition

Some thrive when competing with others
Use it to your advantage
Cultivate friendly competition/support
Desire for Success
Most people have a desire to succeed
Some want success for success' sake
Own it – and reach for your goals
Embrace your desires/No guilt

Money

Some equate money with success
Some just like acquisition: Electronics,
Clothes, Cars, Vacations, Toys,

Food/Housing/Security

If it motivates you, go with it!

Praise

–Some people are motivated because they want
praise
–Also known as recognition/awards/etc.
–Remember to give to others
–Actively seek if it motivates you
–Enter competitions
–Find a path that is rewarded this way

Becoming a better person

Simply wanting to improve who you are
In the workplace
In relationships
Health

Learning
This is particularly strong with internal challenges
Helping others
The desire to do good for others can help you strive to overcome some challenges.
This is a main motivation for some people
If you aren't helping others already, take on the challenge
Find your motivations, use them, and go get your goals!
The view from the top
Those at the top are always seeking to improve and tackle more challenges
It's how they got there to begin with
Must continue to grow if you are going to stay on top
Competition is fierce
Visualize yourself at the top
See yourself reaching your goals
–Where are you?
–What are you wearing?
–What do you look like?
–Who is with you?
–What does it smell like?
–What did you overcome to get here?
Write your goals out and start working on achieving them.
Sometimes the biggest challenge is just getting started
The easiest way is to just start

Now
Not tomorrow
Now!
Once you have started, don't give up
Realize that there will be many, many challenges
See them as opportunities
Keep trying
No matter what
Don't let anything stop you
If you fall down get back up and try again
It isn't failure if you learn from it
Continually identify challenges and actively work
to overcome them
Use the tools above
Remember your motivations

Chapter 8
Calories and you

Once you start to exercise to get some pounds off your body, it is inevitable that you would find yourself weighing yourself on a scale. A tape measure would also be there near you for you to monitor your body measurements. But do you know that it is not only these tools can be used to measure your body mass? It takes you to learn how to count on the calorie intake you have in a day.

Normal calorie intake is 1,200 calories in a day for women and for men, it is around 2,000 calories or a little bit higher than that. There is a difference in counting calories based on different organizations or experts as there are certain factors that need to be considered like age, gender, body build and activity people are involved in.

Nonetheless, if you only take note of proper diet and exercise, you will come to realize that counting the value of your food intake can be just as simple as knowing which food you must not eat and which ones must be found on your table each meal.
If you are on a diet, then, notice what you have been eating. Never let your eyes wander far from what is placed near you. But if you cannot avoid looking at sumptuous delicacies, it's time for you to isolate yourself from the rest of the family to focus on what you must have for the moment. Diet plans have to be strictly followed or else, you'd wind up starting on another program again.

Even if you perform your exercise routines every day and you do not cut back on food, good results are not coming your way. The best solution is to refrain from eating more than what you are required while on a program. Too much exercise to cover up what you have eaten is not a solution that can make you satisfied in the long run.

There are times when a dieter overly does the counting of calories that it results to an adverse situation. Weight loss programs are expected by many as tense on the dieter but only to a point. Such programs can be enjoyable for the dieter and this can be made possible by nutritionists and fitness instructors. These experts can make or break the dreams of their patrons. That is why they take time to give each plan something that the users would easily follow and easily understand.

You may already know that calorie counting is good in the sense that you can grab a hold on your cravings until you have arrived at the weight you are targeting. Too much counting, however, may drive you to paranoia as your mind might be so blinded by the strictness of your routine that you tend to cut back on food intake. You must be aware that you may grow thinner as expected and this is not a good outcome.

To solve this, measure your waist and hips every day and weigh yourself afterwards to see if you are falling short or going overboard your target weight at a given time. In the course of your regimen, you will learn to know which foods are low or high in caloric content.

Being overly eager with the results while in the middle of the program is natural for you as a dieter. But do not get overly excited. You might double your efforts in the gym but this may cause you to become hungrier and consume more than you are allowed to eat. After finding out you have gained instead of losing it, you might fall into a depression. Now, this stress-related problem can make you gobble up a huge quantity of food which eventually would cause you to go back to the basics.

Fiber can be obtained from fruits and vegetables. Both of these types of food are easy to digest and can give you the right nutrients. But as a reminder, fruits contain sugar, too! It is also essential to know the sugar content of each fruit that you will eat to control your blood sugar to a moderate level.

Apart from taking in fiber, you have to understand that there is a need to take in carbohydrates as well as fats. You can burn lots of fats within your system but you still need some to fuel up your rigid activity. Carbohydrates can be avoided but only to a certain level as your body requires it to be there and the control that has to come from you is important.

A cup of raspberries can give you 8.8 grams of fiber and apples of the same quantity can provide you with 4.4 grams. Measure a cup of whole-wheat cooked spaghetti pasta and you'd get 6.3 grams compared to what cooked instant oatmeal can offer which is only around 4 grams. A medium artichoke can offer you 10.3 grams while cooked split peas give out a total of 16.3 grams.

Knowing which fruits and vegetables that can give you more benefits may lead you to become a healthier individual. Just remember that you also have to think about the medical condition you have if there is any in order for you to try on these foods. Some of the foods mentioned may not be good for your condition and might aggravate an illness while you are into a diet program.

Fitness trainers and dietitians know that it is sometimes hard for dieters to understand the meaning of the weight loss phrase. What others simply know is they want to lose weight, they will pay the fee, and they would undergo a series of routines, and wait for results. Understanding what the phrase means can push the dieter to a good start, armed with patience, confidence and trust towards the fitness administrator.

Fat loss and strength training may involve gym equipment to firm up or tone down muscles. Fats can be eliminated just as long as the regimen is religiously followed. Before starting training with equipment, an assessment of the body would ensue and medical records are checked to be sure that there will be no adverse effect on the client.

There are people who envy those who are physically-fit but still go to the gym regularly. The trouble starts when they demand to use some equipment not required of them. This is where excellent trainers come in. These people are knowledgeable on how over eager dieters feel and want to achieve in a short time. Weight loss is not an instant process and every step requires to be performed several times before jumping to the next level.

Diet plans

Skipping meals for the purpose of getting near the target weight and measurement is not a good practice either. For every calorie that is burned, a certain amount of nutrients coming from your food intake is needed to replenish it. So, stick to what your nutritionist has proposed as it will help you a lot in your effort to become slimmer and attractive.

Supplement administration

Supplements may be staples in other gyms but other fitness venues are against it. There are steroids sold to fitness buffs but weight loss patrons may not need it in any way. These add-ons are not for you so stick on your program and benefit from the natural way of eliminating unwanted pounds.

Staying away from eating excessively is an important step you have to take for you to maintain your stand of going along with a weight loss program. Dietitians have known this issue for a long time now and have helped many of their clients overcome the attraction that food brings.

Dieters would laughingly refer to food as evil just because they are not allowed to eat more and calories are counted all the time. But to a certain point, it is just right to stay away from it to help you get your act together and arrive at a good result.

Another blunder that can be a burden is oversleeping. Indeed, some people who are into diet programs will tend to oversleep to make them stay away from their cravings.

This is not good either as the body would tend to relax more and activities that have to be performed along with a planned meal would come to a stoppage. It would be better to sleep 7-8 hours a day, exercise using the right number of minutes, and eat on time with your allowable amount of calories on your plate. As a matter of fact, sleeping helps in weight gain.

Little amounts of liquor and soda can go a long, long way in weight gain if added up within a week's time. If you can avoid bars and pubs, then, try to limit meeting up with your friends who have the habit of passing by these venues right after work. Who says that you can't say no and opt to order orange juice while you see them drinking several rounds of beer? You may not be strong enough to say no when they try all their might to convince you to take a sip. If you can't say no, then avoid that meeting! The same friends that made fun of you, not drinking beer are also the same people that will compliment you when you look better and healthier.

Always remember that you are paying for your diet meal and fitness program. If you can avoid seeing them for a while, do it. Next time they'd see you will be when you have already something to be proud of; but you're not thinking of going back to that vice, right? Even if you are not paying for the weight loss program, let your goal remain in your focus.

Let me include some excerpt from my book "Success is for the ready":

Mental Preparation: *Mental preparation is the first and most important step in succeeding.*

The Key for Success: Success is one hundred percent mental: you have to be mentally prepared for your planned success. Through mental training you will learn how to visualize and imagine your peak performance, and learn how to change negative self-talk and beliefs that are holding you back from performing at your best. Your mental preparedness sits atop of your plan for success. It is this mental toughness that will keep you from folding. Success and failure exist in the power of the mind. Take control of your thoughts and you will take control of your success.

Kick the negatives- the naysayers: *Stay away from people, places, and things that bring you down. Immerse yourself in as many "up building" activities as possible. Choose positive reading material and positive friends. Listen to the utterances of fellow optimists and ignore the criticism of pessimists. Align yourself to a mentor, read articles on persons with dreams similar to yours. Embrace the positives.*

Understand your fears: *Fear creates imaginary obstacles. Fear will prevent you from introducing yourself to people, people who may assist your success (fear of rejection), starting profitable business ventures (fear of failure), and experiencing wonderful things (fear of the unknown). The key to overcoming such fears is to: (a) Recognize them in yourself, (b) identify their root and (c) make a plan to deal with them. Be on the lookout for those who will appear to support your plan, while injecting fear. Should you be hesitant to pursue your dream, ask yourself if fear might be the only thing holding you back? Remove all doubts and fears from your mind and let your plan be materialized. Get beyond your fears and the fears that other people try to give you.*

82

Do not fear failure: *Failure is the spice that gives success its flavor. Success is stumbling from failure to failure with no loss of enthusiasm in the original plan and sometimes, it takes a good fall to really know where you stand in relation to your plan. Although the Wright brothers failed hundreds of times before they succeeded, they never gave up on their dream. If they had, the invention of the modern aircraft would have been credited to someone else. The greatest basket baller of modern times Michael Jordon tells us how many shots he missed in his illustrious career, and the many times he failed to make the one shot that decided the game.*

You cannot fear failure. You must be tenacious and resilient. Each failure means you are one step closer to your goal. Study the failure and determine the cause, solution, and an alternative approach to solving the problem. The people who succeed the most are the people who have failed the most, because they are people who have tried the most. Be patient in failure, The road to success is not to be run upon by swift, but step by step, little by little, bit by bit--that is the way to wealth, that is the way to wisdom, that is the way to glory.

The greatest successes grow out of great failures. In numerous instances the result is better that comes after a series of abortive experiences than it would have been if it had come at once; for all these successive failures induce a skill which is so much additional power working into the final achievement. Every disappointed effort strengthens the base and indicates the only possible path of success, and makes it easier to find.

Persevere: *"Heights that great men reached and kept were not attained by sudden flight, but they while their companions slept were toiling upwards through the night". Keep working toward your goal and tweaking your plan as necessary.*

Think out of the box: *Because it has never been done before does not mean it shouldn't be done. These out of the box successes are the most profound.*

Know Your Limits*: There is a difference between obstacles and limits. Obstacles can be overcome, whereas limits cannot. Real limits are few – obstacles are many. Success is to be measured not so much by the position that one has reached in life as by the obstacles one has overcome while trying to succeed. Knowing your limits will keep you from striving for the unachievable and ending up disappointed. Once you understand your limits, everything outside of them becomes a possibility*
Past successes that have changed the world illustrate the power that exists in the human mind. If our minds have the ability to convince us that something is impossible long before we give it our best effort, If we're not careful, we can formulate a mental surrender that says, "I can't do this. I'll never make it. It's not possible." Those who let themselves think this way are sure to fail because they stop trying to succeed. The Bible says that "As a man thinketh in his heart, so is he" Proverbs 23:7

Chapter 9
Diet Foods

Will power plays an important role for a person who is deprived of something that he can afford to buy.

If you are a cake lover and you are on a diet program, then, you would think that you are on your way to misery. Cry no more as there are solutions to that problem and it is not only you who are facing this dilemma but a lot more people whose aim is just like yours. You are not going to be denied of foods you love to eat until the end of the world. Diet meals can only last for a certain period; after that, you stop and continue with your life, but even when you continue with your life, you must learn to eat the things you love with self-discipline, or you will return to where you started.

The strictness of a diet plan oftentimes drives the dieter to more craving spells than before starting on the program. It would depend on the person if he is able to control the urge to splurge on food that he was denied or turn his back whenever he sees it. But for some people, it doesn't hurt to take a piece as those can be remedied by rigid routines he would perform the next day.

If you like to eat some foods that are not listed on your meal plan, then, go ahead. It wouldn't hurt but promise yourself that you will perform a little bit more active on your next session with your trainer. Depriving you of foods you like to eat may result to cheating all the time. So, grab a bite, savor it until disappears on your throat and lick your lips.

The web can offer you vast solutions to your budget when it comes to finding the right food that you can use on your diet plan. You may either order from a wholesale shop or you can learn to substitute a kind of fruit with another and so as with your vegetable requirements.

Here are some suggestions for you:

Wholesale dealers: Wholesalers offer their products at a lower price compared to retail outlets or are you aware of this? From meat to fruits, straight down to vegetables, prices can be a lot cheaper than you can imagine! Dieters are at awe when it comes to buying from these outlets as they can have the liberty of choosing from available foods to other ingredients they need to cook their own weight loss recipes.

Weight loss websites: There are websites that deal on weight loss that can help teach you how to save on your meal plans. They sometimes offer some ingredients that are hard to find and as long as they are not smelly, they can mail you your orders to your doorstep. Discounts can also be yours once you have gotten lucky on promos on a certain period of time.

Your own backyard: Your own backyard can also be a source for your diet meal recipes. Take a look at what you have. If you don't have any, plant some for the purpose of not going out of your way to travel just for your dinner. Being able to pick some ingredients inside your backyard can be convenient for housewives. You never have to worry about leaving your young kid at home again.

Smoothies as Supplements

Some say that replacing solid meals with smoothies is a good way to achieve ideal weight. But if you are wise enough you must not do so as while smoothies can be nutritious and can offer positive effects towards your aim, they can never replace some nutrients that solid foods bring like protein. There are advantages and disadvantages to the use of this food supplement. Read on to learn about what they constitute and how you can prep yourself up with a nutritious concoction.

- Fats are contained in some smoothie recipes to cover up the need for omega-3. You may use a tablespoonful of oil; in the case of nuts, that would be 2-4 tablespoons. Good suggestions are pistachios, peanut butter, almonds or coconut milk.

- Fruits and veggies are also good ingredients for smoothies. Berries are very nutritious and carb-controlled fruits often used as a staple ingredient in concoctions such as this. Mango, pineapple and bananas are perfect smoothies before and after workouts. Neutral-tasting kale and spinach are ideal fibrous veggies which may turn your smoothie into green but not necessarily affecting its flavor.

- Protein, as an essential part in meals can also be incorporated by using protein powder or the natural blend cottage cheese. Tofu may also serve as an alternative. There are many recipes that use tofu as an ingredient.

- Ice and liquid blended together in a perfect mixture can make a smoothie mouth-watering. Aside from using water, coconut milk or unsweetened almond are ideal. Never add in fruit juices as they contain too much sugar that can hurt your sugar levels. You may adjust your smoothie consistency to your taste.

Keeping Fit by Cooking your Own Meals

What you know about nutritional values in food can make you a successful creator of your own diet meals. Sometimes, it is better to cook your own food rather than buy it cooked from restaurants. You may never know how much oil they use to fry fish or meat and the kind of oil matters to you and your health.

Your diet consists of nutritious ingredients that can make you stand the rigors of exercise and tension during a workout session with a trainer. Your dietitian may draft the best meal for you but the problem is, do you cook meals at home? If so, then, the better for you to save and it is you who can guarantee that you are eating healthy.

Buying all the ingredients from a nearby grocery store if you don't have produce on your backyard by bulk is not advisable. You have to keep your food fresh and a fridge is not a guarantee that you can eat fresh all the time.

Some foods, if frozen can have decreased amount of nutritive value so you have to maintain. Buy for your kitchen foods that you can use within three days if possible. You can purchase whatever you want and cook it as long as it is specified on your meal program.

Follow the instructions your dietitian has specified. To be sure you get the right way of cooking the meal, place a reminder on your fridge's door. So, if your dietitian tells you to cook a certain dish lightly, then, do so.

There is nothing wrong with following instructions to the dot. The only way for you to put on some creativity on your meal is by replacing some ingredients with alternatives that contain the same amount of nutritive value as what has been stated on your guidelines for cooking weight loss recipes.

Growing your Own Diet Foods at Home
Backyard planting is a rising trend and it does not require you much space unless you want to make it big as a breeder or a planter in a metropolitan area! Here are some of the foods that you may find amusing to breed or grow in your backyard that may entail only a period of time but beneficial to you overtime:

Tomatoes: Tomatoes grow on most backyards when taken care of.
Spinach: These green leafy vegetables are easy to grow and can become handy in your backyard whenever you need them.
Even fruit-bearing trees can be planted on pots and this is one of the things that housewives are in favor of. Fruits taken from your backyard are free from toxins brought about by the use of insect sprays and fertilizers.
Okra can easily be planted, green peas and other simple vegetables.

Chapter 10
Nearing the Program's End

What do you think you should do when your weight loss program is nearing its end? Some would say they will rejoice and go to a bar to celebrate while others may invite their friends and party at home. Were you thinking about it too? If you are, then, be prepared to enroll in another program after a couple of months. You will surely become bloated and once again, depression will be knock at your front door.

What does success entail?
Success has lots of different meanings. The most important one is your self-perception. The key to achieving success is believing in yourself and having the strength and motivation to persevere. Success means achieving whatever accomplishments that will keep one from expressing regret when one's final moments come.

Success means being happy with who you are and bringing happiness to those around you. Success means achieving the goal you always dreamed about.

Success is not measured in pride or money, or possessions. It is leading a life that makes you feel proud of yourself and which you bring no harm to others around you.
Success means being able to provide clothing, food, and shelter for those that you bring into this world.
Success is not measured by popularity or money, but with a contented heart.

Achieving your aim or goal is the real definition of success.

Success is having the esteem of one's colleagues.

It would be wiser to celebrate quietly and bask under the splendor of being ogled at by the opposite sex or your colleagues. You will be the central focus of attention; so, be sure you look your best. People who have succeeded in their weight loss programs are considered go-getters and successful individuals as they have experienced a lot of heartaches and patience have become as virtue within themselves. Respect will be yours once you behave like a renewed individual in the eyes of the skeptics.

Party people who have just gone from being heavy to slim may not notice that, taking in a good number of shots at a pub at a given time may immediately give themselves back to their old self. Doing a little bit of restraining your cravings on what used to be your bad habits can offer you more chances of opportunity and this may include refraining from going back to scheduled meals again!

Important Reminders that can Change the Course of your Life
There are a lot of things that you should watch out once you have settled your bill at a fitness gym and your nutritionist. Since there would always be distractions that could lead you to succumb to your past eating habits and boozing, here are some tips that you can utilize and may, perhaps, make you stay away from it all.

- *Choose a new set of friends* - Choosing a new set of friends to go during weekends may give you another chance to widen your horizon. These people may or may not share the same passion as you do but if you know how to look for some aspects where you can start a lengthy conversation with, you just might see something different to talk about. This does not mean making your old friends your enemies, but come on! You know the friends that will pull you back to where you are coming from. Avoid them! Just make them acquaintances.

- *Try a new environment* - You may also opt to relocate to a new environment so you can start fresh. Changing the scenario from metropolitan to a suburb may curb you desire to go bar-hopping and indulging with food. Coping with being overweight isn't just a simple problem that you can easily get away from; it takes you to deal with it at the onset you start looking for food once again that a metropolitan setting can cater you with.

- *Promote a healthy lifestyle* - Promoting a healthy lifestyle is another way to stay away from your former indulgences. Since boozing and excessive eating are what you want to avoid, you can also help others to reclaim their once beautiful bodies by sharing your experiences and how you have overcome obesity; not to mention your addiction to both food and maybe liquor. This way, other people may thank you for opening their eyes to the consequences that these two vices bring.

Regaining your Self-esteem

Obese people have lower self-esteem than lean individuals. Eating is their way of making things look all right even if it isn't so. They would indulge on food and binge on liquor at any chance they see it possible. These people think that they do not need to shed off the pounds they have amassed but instead, decide to stay on with that kind of figure until they start buying maintenance doses for illnesses they have acquired from being fat.

If, for some, fat individuals look happier and satisfied than those with normal weight, then, it is just a façade. People who lack discipline in themselves resort to overindulgence that acts as a mask to protect them from criticisms. What they don't know is those who are there to observe them are already privy to the real situation they are in.

What they feel inside is embarrassment and they also see failure in every effort to take those unsightly bulges on their waists and hips. Now, if they have gotten slim due to a successful weight loss program, there is another dilemma that would beset them and that is regaining self- respect.

Once self-esteem is damaged, it may be hard for you to redeem it lest you have forgotten that you still have some loyal friends left on your side even when the going gets rough. All you need is to muster the remaining amount of confidence left in you to continue prodding yourself into changing what is wrong into right. Staying on what you believe is correct puts back confidence within yourself.

There is definitely a rosy life ahead after a weight loss program. While on it, you might have thought about what if you were not able to make it through all those trying times at the gym and eating foods that you haven't tasted all your life?

Life's sacrifices can ultimately be rewarded by perseverance and the will to change things and also—yourself. It is the brain of the dieter that is the most essential source of all the drive. Look at all resources and motivations placed before you or have been instilled into your mind by able professionals. Use it wisely to topple all negative feelings towards the goal and you wouldn't fail. Unless you want to walk backwards instead of going forward, scheduled programs created for the purpose may pave the way towards a healthier well-being.

Why should you go into the mirror and tell yourself that you do not like to change the way you look? Men and women of today are spending huge sums of money to alter their appearances. So, if you think you can afford to change yours by way of dieting and fitness, and not by any surgery, then, why not? You live in a country that gives you lots of freedom like upgrading your lifestyle and most of all, your body. You can't just walk out of a fitness center and say: "This is too much. I guess I better get going. Bye"!

USE YOUR FREEDOM WISELY

Every determined individual seek to get what he wants. Think about being a finisher rather than a quitter. Where will you go after you have started and eventually called off your program? Are you sure you can face the people whom you have told about your weight loss project? Even if you say that it is you who gets all the pain and pays for your program, people would still look at you with crossed eyebrows. Worst scenario is you may not want to hear what they have to say to you.

Once it enters your mind that you want to see change, then, change it is for you to see. Never rest until you have seen the fruits of your labor. The good outcome of that sacrifice is what may give you satisfaction. Troubles may set in like illnesses and susceptibility to various diseases as your weight rises up on the scale. So, choose between these consequences and the better option.

Socializing can be Fun Again
You will notice that after completing a program that required you to cut back on almost everything, you may look back and think how in the world you have forgotten to love yourself and lived in a life of deprivation just because of life's excesses?
It is not because you have become more successful in life that you can always find a reason to celebrate. It is not because you have money, you can maintain a lot of friends. You have to think that not all of your friends are there to support you anytime; of course, some of them will only be there just because you have the capacity to spend and offer them enjoyment.

Your life is but one and you would wish to spend it as long as you want to live. Your family is more important than people who are not really honest with friendship. You may rethink and reassess your friends by means of telling them that you want to change things. You can always meet up with them but not to the point of re-enjoying the night with all the excesses you used to share.

Real friends would always understand what you meant by that and they will learn to love you more. If you are brave enough to tell them that you want to change your life for the better by means of staying away from booze or excessive eating, then, you may do so any time you want to start it with. Accept the fact that you are in another phase of your life and this is not only for your own good but for the rest of the people who love you.

Thank you so much for reading my book. If I brought some inspiration to you, why not email me at support@janejohn-nwankwo.com?

Please check out and buy my other titles. I have published 50 books as at date.

My website is www.janejohn-nwankwo.com

ABOUT THE AUTHOR

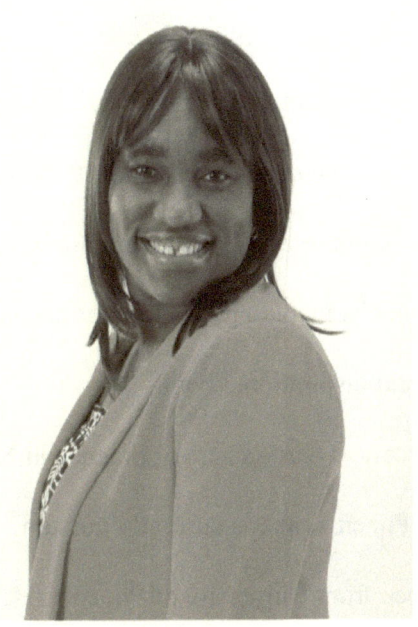

Jane John-Nwankwo CPT, RN, MSN, PHN is a motivational speaker and published author of more than 45 books which include textbooks for healthcare training, fiction for entertainment, how to start small businesses, and motivational books.
Simply search
"Books by Jane John-Nwankwo"
On Amazon.com, Barnes & Nobles, etc

Visit her website:
www.janejohn-nwankwo.com

Book Jane John-Nwankwo as your motivational speaker

now at www.JaneJohn-Nwankwo.com

With more than 10 years as a professional speaker, Jane John-Nwankwo can hold any audience sitting straight on their chairs for any length of time! She is a published author of more than 45 books including "It's in your hands" (A motivational and inspirational book)

She received her Masters of Science in Nursing from University of Phoenix, and is currently pursuing a PhD in Nursing Science from University of Phoenix. Her speaking interests include: Motivational speeches for new business owners, Motivational speeches for any category of people, Employee seminars, Students' Empowerment, Healthcare topics, Topics related to women, and any Christian topic. Book a speaking appointment today and become a repeat customer because of 100% satisfaction.

OTHER TITLES FROM THE SAME AUTHOR:

1. Hightime you made a move!

2. Accept challenges

3. Never be intimidated

4. Design your own methods to navigate

5. Success is for the ready

6. How to market a website

7. How to start your own business

8. How to make money online with no money

Have you bought these books?

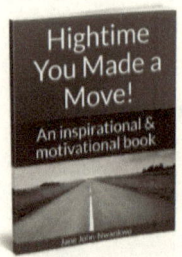 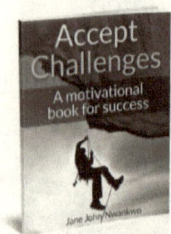 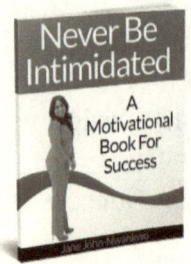

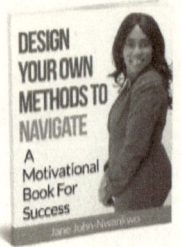 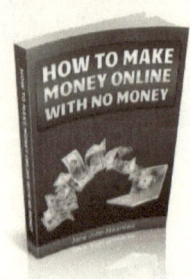 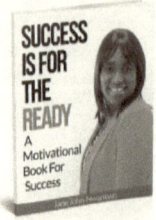

www.ingramcontent.com/pod-product-compliance
Lightning Source LLC
Chambersburg PA
CBHW021210290526
45796CB00005B/28